CARB CYCLING FOR WEIGHT LOSS

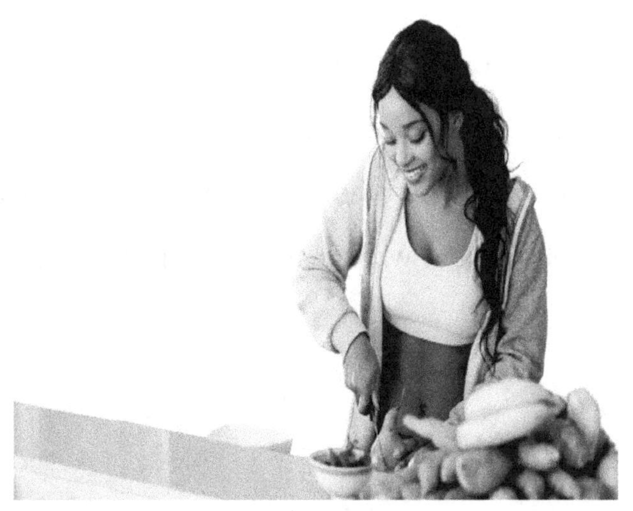

The Ultimate Guide to Carb Cycling for Rapid Weight Loss with Exercise Recipes and Meal plans.

Aspect J. Victory

Table of Contents

INTRODUCTION

Chapter 1: What is Carb Cycling?

Benefits of Carb Cycling for Weight Loss:

- How carb cycling promotes weight loss

Chapter 2: The Science Behind Carb Cycling

- Research on the effectiveness of carbohydrate cycling.

Chapter 3: Understanding Macronutrients

- Designing a balanced meal for carbohydrate cycling

Chapter 4: Getting Started with Carb Cycling

Chapter 5: Basic Carb Cycling on the Right Foot

Chapter 6: Meal Planning and Recipes

- Sample recipes for carb cycling days.

Chapter 7: Exercise and Carb Cycling

- The importance of exercise.

Chapter 8: Monitoring Progress and Tracking Results

Chapter 9: Common Questions and Concerns

- Addressing FAQs about Carb Cycling

- Dealing with Challenges and Misconceptions

Chapter 10: Conclusion and Next Steps

- Moving Forward with Carb Cycling for Continued Success

INTRODUCTION

Emily was an avid reader and she always looked for new knowledge and inspiration in the pages of books. But despite her love of reading, she struggled with her weight and felt discouraged by failed attempts at following a traditional diet. One rainy afternoon, while browsing in a dusty old bookstore, Emily came across a worn volume titled "The Science of Nutrition and Fitness." Intrigued, she bought the book and passionately delved into its pages.

As she flipped through the chapters, Emily came across a concept she had never heard of before: carb cycling.

The book explains how alternating between high and low carbohydrate intake can optimize fat loss while maintaining muscle mass. Emily was intrigued by this novel approach and decided to give it a try.

Armed with new knowledge, Emily meticulously created a nutrition plan based on the principles of carb cycling. On high-carb days, she indulged in healthy grains, fruits and vegetables and fueled her body for intense workouts. On low-carb days, she relied on lean protein, healthy fats, and fiber-rich vegetables to keep her energy levels stable.

To her surprise, Emily began to see results. The pounds melted away and she felt more energetic and confident than ever. As the weeks turned into months, her friends and family noticed her transformation.

News of Emily's success spread throughout the city and she was soon inundated with requests for advice and guidance. Inspired by her own journey, Emily decided to share her knowledge with others, hosting workshops and creating online resources to help people achieve their health and fitness goals through carb cycling.

Thanks to Emily's innovation and determination, carb cycling became a widely used method for weight loss and body transformation. And as Emily remembered her journey, she realized that sometimes the most extraordinary discoveries are found in the pages of a simple book.

Welcome to Carb Cycling for Weight Loss, a complete guide to understanding and implementing the powerful carb cycling strategy for effective weight loss. If she struggles with traditional diet methods or finds it difficult to maintain long-term results, carb cycling for weight loss offers a flexible and sustainable approach that can transform her relationship with food and her body.

In recent years, carb cycling has gained popularity among fitness enthusiasts, athletes, and people looking for a balanced, manageable way to lose excess weight while optimizing their energy levels and performance. Unlike restrictive diets that require constant deprivation, carb cycling allows for strategic manipulation of carbohydrate intake, providing the body with the fuel it needs while promoting fat loss and maintaining muscle mass.

In this book, we delve into the science behind carb cycling and explore how it affects metabolism, hormonal regulation, and overall body composition. You'll gain a deeper understanding of how different macronutrients affect your energy levels, your cravings, and your ability to burn fat, allowing you to make informed decisions about your eating habits.

But "Carb Cycling for Weight Loss" is more than just a collection of scientific theories. It's a practical roadmap designed to help you easily navigate the complexities of carb cycling. Whether you're a beginner looking to jump-start your weight loss journey or a seasoned fitness enthusiast looking to perfect your approach, this book offers step-by-step instructions, customizable meal plans, and expert advice to ensure your success.

On these pages you will discover:
- The basics of carb cycling and how it differs from traditional dietary approaches.
– The science behind carbohydrate metabolism and its role in energy production and fat storage.
- Strategies to determine your individual carb cycling needs based on factors such as activity level, body composition, and goals.
- Practical tips for meal planning, shopping and preparing delicious, nutritious meals that will help you lose weight.
- Guidance for overcoming common challenges and setbacks, including food cravings, plateaus, and social situations.
- Try workout routines and exercise recommendations to complement your carb cycling protocol and maximize your results.

As you embark on this journey, remember that sustainable weight loss is not about deprivation or extreme measures. It's about finding a balanced approach that nourishes your body, fuels your training, and supports your overall well-being. With the knowledge and tools provided in this book, you will be able to adopt carb cycling as a lifestyle, paving the way for long-term success and radiant health.

Are you ready to transform your body and revolutionize your approach to weight loss? Let's start the journey together.

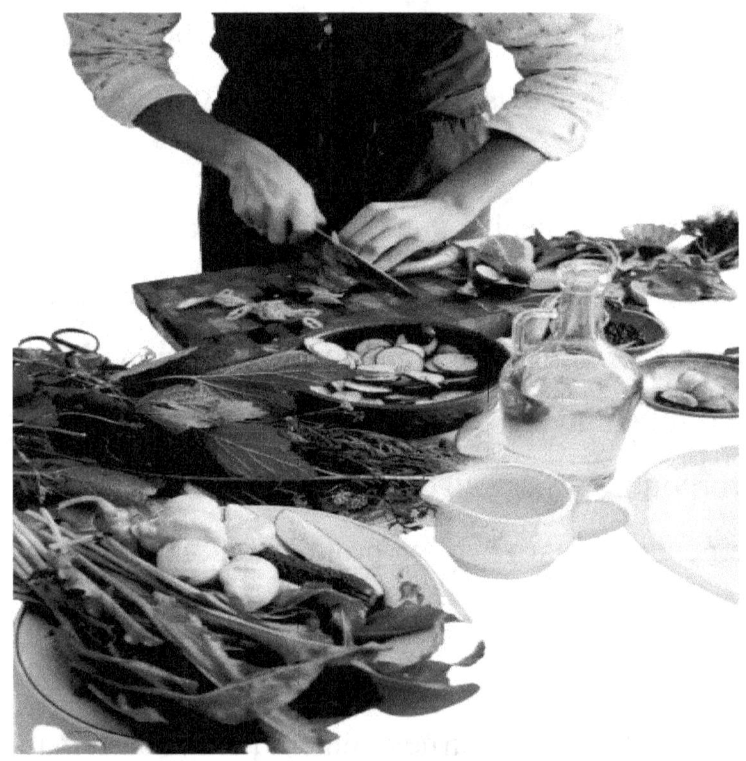

Chapter 1: What is Carb Cycling?

Carbohydrates, sometimes called carbs, are an ongoing hot topic now. Some nutritional experts are starting to associate them with problems such as inflammation, diabetes and obesity. However, others continue to insist that they are an essential part of our daily diet.

So are all carbohydrates bad for you? And how many carbohydrates should you eat every day? Carb cycling help this way

Carb cycling is a nutritional strategy that varies the amount of carbohydrates consumed on a daily or weekly basis. Instead of sticking to a consistent carb intake every day, alternate between high-carb days, medium-carb days, and low-carb days. The goal is to strategically manage carbohydrate consumption to meet energy needs, promote fat loss, and improve performance during exercise.

Carbohydrates, along with fat and protein, make up the three macronutrients. When your body digests carbohydrates, they are broken down into glucose - your brain and body's preferred form of energy. When glucose enters the bloodstream, the pancreas is triggered to produce a hormone called insulin. Glucose transporter proteins are responsible for transporting glucose from the bloodstream into the cell. Here it is converted into energy, stored in the fat cells or stored as glycogen.

Choosing a high-carb diet can help you reduce body fat while increasing muscle mass. Since this is an extremely strict diet, it should only be used for a short period of time. However, it is useful for breaking through weight loss plateaus.

Carb cycling involves increasing and decreasing carbohydrate intake on different days of the week. There are high-carb days and low-carb days, as well as days when no carbohydrates are eaten at all. If you try carb cycling, you can eat carbohydrates if they come from a clean source. Cycling allows the body to use fat as fuel more effectively, rather than burning muscle tissue and carbohydrates.

Benefits of Carb Cycling for Weight Loss:

Carb cycling is not ideal for everyone. However, under the right circumstances, it can prove to be a useful solution. There are two main groups of people who can benefit from trying this diet: those who need to lose weight and those who want to build muscle mass while increasing their athletic performance.

Do I have to lose weight?

Some experts say carb cycling is particularly beneficial for anyone who needs to lose weight. In theory, this type of diet can help maintain physical performance. It also offers many of the same benefits that low-carb diets like the Atkins diet offer. Such diets can leave dieters feeling lethargic and weak. Therefore, carb cycling provides a distinct advantage..

Like any other diet, the main mechanism for losing weight is to maintain a calorie deficit. you have to eat less.

There is more food than the body can burn over a long period of time. Anyone who switches to carbohydrate intake at the same time as a calorie deficit will almost certainly lose weight.

Carbs are not bad for you. However, the function of carbohydrates is to provide your body with a source of energy to burn when you are active. If you don't exercise enough and still eat a lot of carbohydrates, problems arise. Ultimately, your body stores the excess as fat.

Carbohydrates are a good option when you train hard in the gym. Your body will burn them quickly to create energy. It burns carbohydrates instead of protein, so this nutrient can stimulate muscle growth.

If you don't train hard, these extra carbs won't be burned off quickly. Therefore, the body stores all unused glucose in fat cells. This leads to overweight or even obesity.

On the other hand, if you limit your carbohydrate intake, your body will not be able to store excess glucose. Instead, fats are used for energy instead of starchy or sugary foods. This allows your body to break down fat, which helps you lose weight.

If you have a very active lifestyle, it's perfectly okay to consume extra calories. However, if you don't exercise a lot, you won't be able to consume all of your calories. This leads to obesity. Therefore, it is necessary to vary carbohydrate intake from day to day. Going to the gym can help you consume more carbohydrates. If you watch television most of the day, you may want to consider limiting your consumption.

Another reason carb cycling is so good for weight loss is that it makes it harder to overeat. Foods rich in carbohydrates tend to be tastier. We all know how hard it is to resist the temptation of eating another cookie or a delicious sugary donut. It is much more difficult to eat excessive amounts of vegetables and protein. Very few people eat too much chicken or broccoli!

This will help you burn fewer calories and improve your waistline.

Because carb cycling is a flexible way to diet, it may be more appealing to dieters. Knowing that you can occasionally consume carbohydrates can be attractive. One of the reasons so many people fail with other diets is their restrictive nature. Knowing that you will never be able to eat pasta or bread can be discouraging from the beginning. This causes dieters to give up after a short period of time. The flexibility of carb cycling may encourage these people to stick with the program. As a result, they lose more weight overall and maintain a healthier body weight.

There is also an important connection between blood insulin levels and carbohydrate intake. If blood insulin levels are high, fat is more likely to be stored. This, in turn, makes effective weight loss difficult. You should be careful to modify your carbohydrate intake when taking insulin for diabetes.

Consulting a medical professional is crucial.

Healthy eating should also be at the center of any carb cycling plan. It is not an excuse to restrict eating habits to excessive levels or to abuse unhealthy foods. Successful carb cycling requires careful monitoring. This can promote unhealthy attitudes toward food. That is why you must be careful and aware of everything when introducing this regimen. If you find that it is having a negative impact

When you change your life in this way, you need to stop and choose a different eating plan.

Implement carb cycling

High carb days

On high-carb days, you should aim for 2 to 2.5 grams of carbs per pound of body weight. These days tend to coincide with your most intense training days, as higher carbohydrate intake can fuel your training and stimulate insulin release, which promotes nutrient delivery and glycogen replenishment.

Low carb days

On low-carb days, aim for 0.5 grams of carbs per pound of body weight. These days are usually rest days or low intensity training days. Lower carbohydrate intake promotes fat loss and increases insulin sensitivity.

Days without carbs

Carb-free days are often included in more advanced carb cycling plans. These days, try to eat less than 30 grams of carbohydrates a day. This can help further promote fat loss and increase insulin sensitivity.

Example of a carb cycling plan

Below is an example of a carb cycling plan for someone who trains five days a week:

Monday: high carbs

Tuesday: low carb

Wednesday: high carb

Thursday: low carb

Friday: high carb

Saturday: No carbs

Sunday: low carb

food to eat

On high-carb days, focus on eating complex carbs like sweet potatoes, brown rice, quinoa, oats, and fruit. On low-carb and no-carb days, focus on lean proteins, non-starchy vegetables, and healthy fats.

- How carb cycling promotes weight loss

Carb cycling is a nutritional approach that involves alternating between high- and low-carb days throughout the week. Due to its potential to promote fat loss while maintaining muscle mass, it has become very popular among fitness enthusiasts and those looking to lose weight. Understanding how the carbohydrate cycle works and the effects it has on the body can shed light on why it is effective for weight loss.

In essence, carb cycling manipulates carbohydrate absorption to optimize fat burning while simultaneously providing the body with the energy it needs for physical activity. On high-carbohydrate days, people consume more carbohydrates, usually from sources such as whole grains, fruits, and starchy vegetables. These carbohydrates replenish glycogen stores in the muscles and liver, providing energy for intense workouts and daily activities. This increased carbohydrate intake also helps stimulate insulin secretion, which promotes muscle growth and recovery.

On the other hand, low carb days involve reducing your carbohydrate intake and often relying more on protein and healthy fats for energy. By restricting carbohydrate intake, the body is forced to rely on stored fat for fuel, which increases fat burning. This metabolic shift can help people overcome weight loss plateaus and accelerate fat loss, especially when combined with regular exercise.

One of the main benefits of carb cycling for weight loss lies in its ability to prevent metabolic adaptation, a phenomenon in which the body adjusts its metabolic rate in response to sustained caloric restriction or low carbohydrate intake. Prolonged calorie deficits or strict low-carb diets can cause a decrease in metabolic rate over time, making it increasingly difficult to continue losing weight. Carb cycling avoids this problem by reintroducing carbohydrates into the diet at regular intervals. This signals to the body that energy resources are abundant and the metabolic rate should remain elevated. This proactive approach helps prevent metabolism slowing and maintain a more efficient fat burning environment in the body. Additionally, carb cycling offers a level of flexibility and sustainability that is often missing in more strict nutritional approaches. Unlike crash low-carb diets, which can be difficult to follow long-term due to their restrictive nature, carb cycling allows you to enjoy high-carb meals on a regular basis without sacrificing progress. This flexibility not only improves diet compliance, but also makes socializing and eating out easier, as people can enjoy occasional treats without feeling guilty or disrupting their overall eating plan.

Additionally, carb cycling can be tailored to individual preferences, goals, and lifestyles. Some people may benefit from more frequent high-carbohydrate days, especially if they engage in vigorous physical activity or have higher energy needs due to factors such as a physically demanding job. Conversely, others may find success with a low-carb approach, with fewer high-carb days and a greater emphasis on fat adaptation and ketosis.

In short, carb cycling is a multipronged approach to weight loss that uses the body's response to different amounts of carbohydrates to optimize fat burning, preserve muscle mass, and prevent metabolic adaptation. By strategically alternating between high- and low-carb days, people can create a sustainable and effective nutritional program that supports their weight loss goals while allowing flexibility, enjoyment, and long-term compliance. When combined with regular exercise and mindful eating habits, carb cycling can be a valuable tool for improving body composition and overall health.

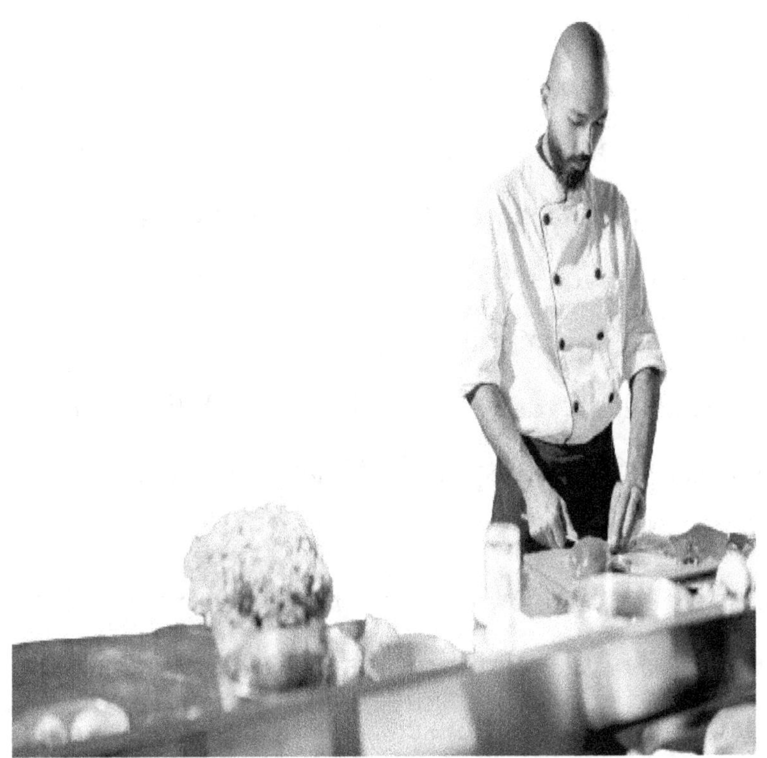

Chapter 2: The Science Behind Carb Cycling

Surely! Let's delve into the fascinating world of carbohydrate cycling and explore the science behind this nutritional strategy. Whether you're an athlete, fitness enthusiast, or simply interested in optimizing your diet, understanding carbohydrate cycling can help you make informed decisions.

The science behind carb cycling

The science behind carb cycling lies in its ability to manipulate insulin and metabolic response. Is that how it works:

insulin sensitivity

insulin is a hormone produced by the beta cell cells of the pancreas One of the main benefits of carb cycling is the potential to improve insulin sensitivity. On low carb days, your body is more sensitive to insulin and can do its job more efficiently.

metabolic advantage

Carb cycling can also create a "metabolic advantage" by alternating between high and low carb days. This variation may prevent the slowing of metabolism that often accompanies prolonged periods of calorie restriction.

Burning fat

On low carb days, carb cycling aims to increase fat burning. Without an adequate supply of glucose and glycogen (which will be depleted over the course of your low-carb and fasting days), your body is forced to adapt and rely on an energy source that is available: the fat stored in your cells. .

Implement carb cycling

Implementing a carb cycling plan can be relatively easy. Here's a basic weekly setup:

Monday: high carbs

Tuesday: low carb

Wednesday: high carb

Thursday: low carb

Friday: high carb

Saturday: low carb

Sunday: No carbs

Remember, high-carb days should correspond with your most intense training days, while low-carb days should correspond with rest days or low-intensity training days.

Diploma

Carb cycling is a flexible diet strategy that can be tailored to individual goals, whether that's losing weight, building muscle, or improving performance. Although carb cycling has its benefits, it is not necessary for everyone. This is just one method that can help some people better manage their diet and achieve their health and fitness goals.

Remember that the most important factor in any diet is adherence. The best diet for you is one that you can follow long term. Always consult a doctor or registered dietitian before starting a new diet or exercise program.

Carbohydrate Cycling: A Deeper Insight

The role of hormones

Carb cycling can have profound effects on your body's hormones. Understanding this will help you maximize effectiveness.

leptin

Leptin is a hormone produced by fat cells in the body. It is often referred to as the "satiety hormone" or the "hunger hormone." The main target of leptin is in the brain, specifically in an area called the hypothalamus. Leptin is designed to tell your brain that if you have enough fat stored, you don't need to eat and that you can burn calories normally. Carb cycling can help keep leptin levels balanced, preventing the crash that can occur when dieting.

ghrelin

Ghrelin is often referred to as the "hunger hormone." When your stomach is empty, it releases ghrelin and sends a signal to the brain to trigger the feeling of hunger. Interestingly, ghrelin levels can be reduced during times of low carbohydrate intake, helping to alleviate feelings of hunger during those times.

Carbohydrate cycling and sports performance

Carbohydrate cycling can also be a useful strategy for athletes who want to optimize their performance. By combining high-carbohydrate days with high-intensity training days, athletes can ensure their bodies have the fuel they need to perform at their best. Low and no carb days can be combined with rest days or low intensity training days.

Possible disadvantages of carb cycling

While carb cycling can be an effective way to lose weight and improve performance, it is not without its potential drawbacks.

These may include:

Complexity: Carb cycling requires a lot of planning and nutritional knowledge to do correctly.

Possible nutrient deficiency: If carbohydrate cycling is not properly planned, deficiencies of certain nutrients may occur, particularly fiber and certain vitamins.

Potential for eating disorders: The strict nature of carbohydrate cycling could potentially lead to unhealthy eating behaviors in some people.

Diploma

Carb cycling is a powerful tool in the right hands, but it's not for everyone. To be effective, a good knowledge of nutrition and careful planning are required. As always, it is recommended to consult a doctor or registered dietitian before beginning any new diet or exercise program. It's also important to remember that while diet plays a crucial role in health and fitness, it is only one piece of the puzzle. Regular exercise, adequate sleep, and stress management are also important parts of a healthy lifestyle.

- Research on the effectiveness of carbohydrate cycling.

Research on the effectiveness of carbohydrate cycling requires a multifaceted examination of its potential advantages and disadvantages in different contexts. This nutritional strategy, characterized by alternating periods of high and low carbohydrate intake, has generated significant interest in the areas of weight control, optimization of sports performance, and improvement of metabolic health.

Studies examining the effects of carbohydrate cycling typically address several key areas. First, researchers are studying its effectiveness in promoting weight or fat loss compared to traditional continuous carbohydrate intake regimens. This includes analyzing changes in body composition, metabolic markers and overall energy balance over longer periods of time.

Additionally, the effects of carbohydrate cycling on athletic performance are being closely examined. Athletes and fitness enthusiasts use carbohydrate cycling to manipulate glycogen stores and optimize energy levels for training and competition. Research efforts are aimed at determining whether periodic carbohydrate restriction followed by refueling produces performance benefits such as increased endurance, strength, or recovery.

Metabolic health parameters are also examined in carbohydrate cycling studies. Studies could focus on its influence on insulin sensitivity, blood sugar control, lipid profiles and inflammatory markers. It is critical to understand how carbohydrate cycling affects metabolic health, particularly in populations predisposed to insulin resistance, metabolic syndrome, or type 2 diabetes.

Additionally, the nuances of carbohydrate cycling are carefully examined, including variations in carbohydrate intake, timing, and individual responsiveness. Researchers strive to identify optimal carbohydrate cycling protocols tailored to specific goals, metabolic profiles, and lifestyle preferences.

Despite its potential benefits, there is no general agreement on the effectiveness of carb cycling. Study results often provide conflicting results and highlight the complexity of nutritional interventions and individual variability in responses. Factors such as participant characteristics, study duration, compliance with prescribed protocols, and methodological considerations contribute to the heterogeneity of research results.

In summary, ongoing research efforts aim to deepen our understanding of the effectiveness of carbohydrate cycling in various areas. By elucidating its effects on weight management, athletic performance, and metabolic health, scientists aim to refine nutritional recommendations and optimize personalized nutritional strategies for different populations..

Chapter 3: Understanding Macronutrients

Understanding macronutrients

Macronutrients are nutrients that your body needs in large quantities to function properly. These include carbohydrates, proteins and fats. Each of these macronutrients plays a critical role in your body's health and well-being. Understanding these macronutrients is important, especially when considering a nutritional strategy like carb cycling for weight loss.

carbohydrates

Carbohydrates are the body's main source of energy. They are broken down into glucose, which the body uses as an energy source for the muscles and brain. Simple and Complex are the 2 primary category of Carbohydrates. Simple carbohydrates or sugars give your body a quick burst of energy, while complex carbohydrates or starches provide long-lasting energy.

When carb cycling, there are days when you eat more carbs and days when you eat less. The idea is to meet the body's energy needs without overwhelming it, which can lead to weight gain.

Proteins

Proteins are the building blocks of your body. They are used to build and repair tissues, produce enzymes and hormones and are essential for forming bones, muscles, cartilage, skin and blood. Like carbohydrates, protein can be used for energy, but the body primarily uses it for growth and repair.

Protein is especially important on low-carb days in a carb cycling plan. It helps maintain muscle mass and provides a feeling of satiety, which can be helpful when losing weight.

Fats

Fats are a concentrated source of energy. Your body needs them for growth and development, vitamin absorption, inflammation, and regulation of blood clotting and brain function. There are various types of fats, such as , trans, unsaturated and saturated fats.

Healthy fats also play a crucial role in a carb cycling diet. On low carb days, fats become the main source of energy. It's important to choose healthy fats, such as those found in avocados, nuts, seeds, and olive oil, rather than unhealthy fats, such as those found in fried foods and baked goods.

The role of macronutrients in the carbohydrate cycle.

When carb cycling, the balance of these macronutrients changes depending on the day. On high-carb days, your diet will be high in carbs and protein, but low in fat. On low carb days, your diet will be high in protein and fat but low in carbs. The idea behind carb cycling is to maximize the body's energy consumption and improve metabolic processes. By varying your macronutrient intake, you can better control your blood sugar levels, manage your weight, and improve your overall health.

Diploma

Understanding macronutrients and their role in the body is crucial when considering a diet like carb cycling. By knowing what each macronutrient does and how to balance them, you can create a diet plan that will help you lose weight, maintain muscle mass, and improve your health.

Remember that while diet is a crucial part of weight loss and health, it is only one piece of the puzzle. Regular exercise, adequate sleep, and stress management are also important for achieving and maintaining a healthy weight. Always consult a doctor or registered dietitian before starting a new diet or exercise program.

- Designing a balanced meal for carbohydrate cycling

Developing a balanced carb cycling nutrition plan requires strategic manipulation of carbohydrate intake to optimize energy levels and support specific fitness goals. Carb cycling typically involves alternating high and low carb days to increase fat loss, muscle retention, and performance.
Here is a complete guide to creating balanced meals for carb cycling:

Understand the phases of the carbohydrate cycle:
High carbohydrate days: These days are characterized by increased carbohydrate intake, usually associated with intense workouts to increase performance and promote muscle glycogen replenishment.

Low Carb Days: On these days, carbohydrate intake is reduced to encourage the body to use stored fat as an energy source, promoting fat loss and metabolic flexibility.

Determine daily calorie needs:

To calculate your total daily energy expenditure (TDEE), consider the following: health, activity level, weight, goals and age.

Adjust your calorie intake depending on whether you want to lose fat, maintain weight, or build muscle.

Allocate carbohydrates:

On high-carb days, allocate a greater percentage of your total calorie intake to carbohydrates, usually around 45-65% of your total calories.

On low-carb days, reduce your carbohydrate intake to approximately 10 to 30 percent of your total calories.

Focus on complex carbohydrates:

On high-carb days, prioritize complex carbohydrates to provide sustained energy and support muscle recovery.

Examples include whole grains, sweet potatoes, quinoa, and legumes.

Include lean protein sources:

Incorporate lean protein sources into every meal to support muscle repair and growth. Opt for options like chicken breast, turkey, fish, tofu, tempeh, eggs, and low-fat dairy.

Incorporate healthy fats:

Eat healthy fats in moderation to support hormone production, satiety, and overall health. Sources include avocado, nuts, seeds, olive oil, and fatty fish such as salmon.

Prioritize foods rich in fiber:

Choose fiber-rich vegetables and fruits to increase satiety, aid digestion, and regulate blood sugar levels. Examples include leafy greens, broccoli, berries, and apples.

Adjust portion sizes:

Adjust portion sizes to individual calorie and macronutrient needs. Ensure adequate protein intake to support muscle maintenance or growth, especially on low-carb days.

Drink enough:

Hydration is essential for overall health and performance. Drink plenty of water throughout the day, especially during exercise and in hot weather.

Time to eat:

Schedule your carbohydrate intake around training to optimize performance and recovery. Consume higher levels of carbohydrates before and after exercise to stimulate activity and replenish glycogen stores.

Listen to your body:

Pay attention to how your body reacts to different amounts of carbohydrates and adjust your eating plan accordingly. The need and tolerance for carbohydrates may be different for each person.

Consult a professional:

If you are unsure how to create a carb cycling eating plan or have specific dietary concerns, consult a registered dietitian or nutritionist to tailor a plan to your individual needs and goals.een high-carb and low-carb days to enhance fat loss, muscle retention, and performance.

Chapter 4: Getting Started with Carb Cycling

Although the idea of carb cycling is appealing, it's hard to know how to get started. This type of diet can be quite complex. Therefore, it is necessary to know as much as possible about carbohydrates and how they work in the body. Additionally, it's crucial to possess an understanding of the principles involved in selecting the optimal carb cycling approach that aligns with your specific needs and goals.

The information we have provided in previous chapters will help you find the right program for you. However, you could probably benefit from some expert advice to help you get off to a good start. Here are some good tips to point you in the right direction.

First, let's look at how we can avoid the biggest drawbacks of carb cycling. Here are some of the most common:

Focus solely on carbs and ignore other macros.: Carb cycling is not just about carbs. It's about balancing your calorie intake throughout the week. When carbohydrate intake is reduced on a rest day, more protein and fat must be consumed to compensate. This is the only way to maintain long-term fat loss.

First you need to know how many calories you need to consume to maintain your weight. This allows you to plan the amount you need to adapt your intake to each day of rest or training. On a rest day, reduce 10 to 20 percent of your calorie intake from carbohydrates, but don't increase your protein or fat intake. Each gram of carbohydrate contains four calories. If you consume a thousand calories a day, reduce your carbohydrate intake by 50 grams on rest days.

Your calorie intake fluctuates too much. The 10 to 20 percent rule applies specifically to carbohydrates. However, the difference in the total number of calories you consume throughout the week should never be more than 33 percent. Too much variation impairs recovery. It also makes it difficult to maintain the carbohydrate pacing regimen. You can remedy this by consuming at least 68 percent of your usual energy intake on low-carb days.

You use your high carb days as a cheat day.: High performance days are no reason to eat everything you like. If you do this regularly, unhealthy eating habits will begin to develop. You can solve this problem by focusing mainly on nutrient-dense foods.

Eat more whole foods like oats and potatoes on your high-carb days.: Eat more nuts and eggs on your low carb days. You'll feel full, but it won't ruin your overall diet.

Now that you know what to avoid, here are some tips for any carb cycling program.

Base the nutritional approach you choose on your activity level and initial caloric needs.

Choose your refeed days well in advance. Always follow your regimen until the day of refeeding.

Make all your decisions based on the result.

Different renutrition strategies work best for different body types. To make sure you are on the best path for you, you should take body composition tests.

Exercise on your refeed days.: This ensures the best body composition results. On refeeding days, eat more carbohydrates in the morning and during times when you are doing a lot of physical activity.

Eat more leafy greens on low-carb days. They are practically calorie-free, but they add more volume to your plate. You will find that a full-looking dish will be more satisfying.

Eat whole fats on low-carb days. Cold water fish, nuts, grass-fed butter, eggs, avocado, and coconut oil are good options.

Measure your carbohydrates and fats. This allows you to track how many calories you consume. On a normal day, measure your carbohydrates as well. We often underestimate the amount of protein we eat and overestimate the amount of fat and carbohydrates.

Don't reduce your carbohydrate intake without eating more fat. Your body needs fats or carbohydrates for energy. This means you need to energize yourself for the day in one way or another.

Avoid skipping meals. You may be tempted to skip meals on regular or low-carb days to lose more weight. That's a bad idea. This could cause your body to break down more muscles.

Avoid improvising. The decision to try carb cycling is very different from reality. You must be dedicated and keep detailed records of your intake at each meal. You have to do this every day for weeks. There is no way to look at an ingredient and determine its calorie and macronutrient content. Therefore, you must measure and record accordingly. Apps like MyPlate and My Fitness Pal are suitable for this.

Always choose foods that support your overall well-being, even on high-carb days. Large amounts of pasta and white bread, liters of sugary drinks and a lot of cake are not exactly good for your health.   Here are carbohydrates complex that are higher in fiber Quinoa, whole wheat bread, and oats are filling and filling. They have numerous benefits.

Treat yourself from time to time.: Just because you should eat healthy most of the time doesn't mean you can never indulge. If you forbid yourself from eating desserts or bagels, you'll end up craving them. The result is that you end up cheating even more and ruining your diet. It could also lead to an unhealthy relationship with food and eating over time. If you opt for complex carbohydrates on most high-carb days, you can eat the occasional cookie or chocolate bar.

Talk to an expert.: Nutrition can be a complex and nuanced topic for everyone. Therefore, working closely with a professional could be a good idea. A nutritionist can create an individual nutrition plan tailored to your needs. It adapts to your specifications, your goals and your activity level. This

ensures that you get all the right nutrients and still get the
results you want.

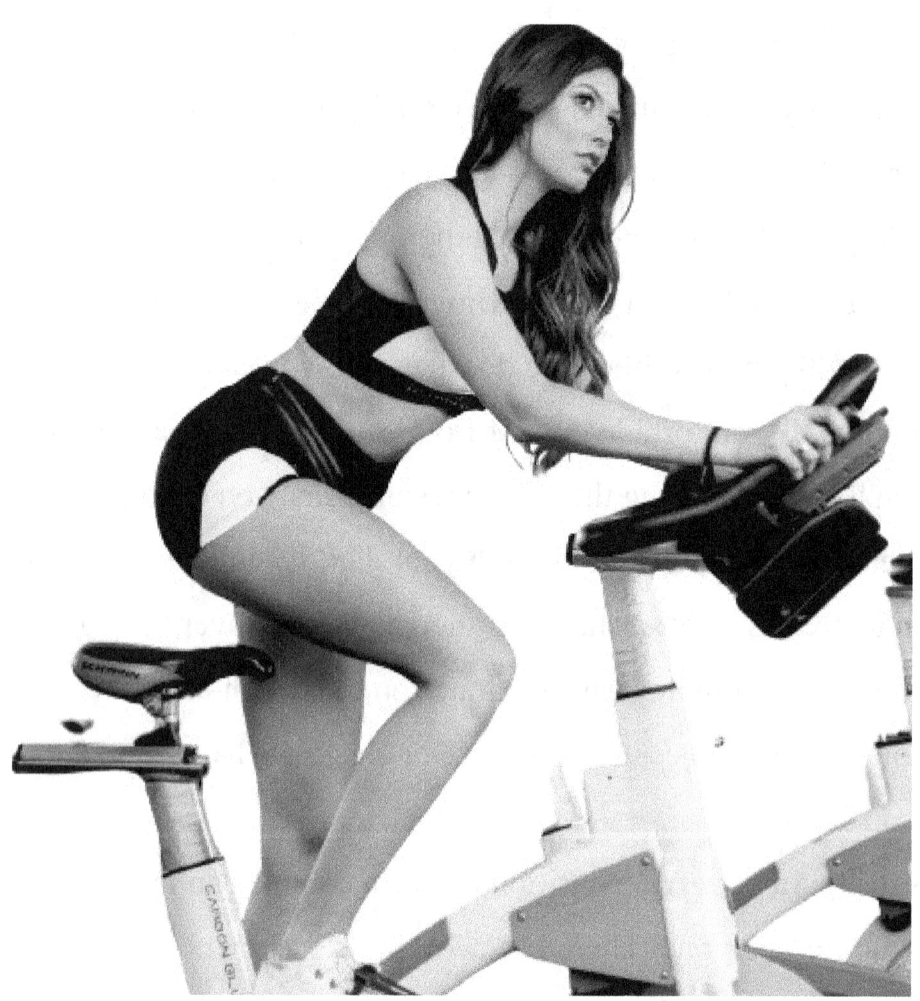

Chapter 5: Basic Carb Cycling on the Right Foot

A little preparation before starting your plan will save you a lot of time, hassle, and mistakes. These are the basics you need to get started on the right foot.

Choose your plan

First, decide which days will be your high carb days and which will be your low carb days. For convenience, we use the alternating high and low carb daily schedule. If you want to use another version described above, simply change the meal plans to fit your days.

Ideally, your high-carb days should correspond to the days when you are most active. However, this is not a rule. Next, choose your "cheat day."

This is the plan you will follow for the next month. It is not recommended to change plans mid-course as this would break the existing cycle.

Set the number of meals

The number of meals you eat per day depends entirely on you. Some people prefer four to six smaller meals instead of the traditional three. This type of plan might be right for you if you're used to snacking more throughout the day. The 3-meal plans also include healthy snacks. If you are the type of person who is often hungry, it is better to eat more meals a day. More advanced carb cyclers may include fasting or eating only two meals a day. Although it may seem appealing, this approach is strongly discouraged for individuals with limited experience.

Establish the meal plan for your week

That's the fun part! It's best to plan your meals weekly, biweekly, or even monthly if you're really organized. This saves you the hassle of preparing a meal at the last minute. The meal plan should indicate the day, whether it is high or low carbohydrate, and the number of meals.

After each meal, you must indicate the time at which you will eat it. The times are just a general framework. On days when you are hungry, you can eat your next meal a little earlier. There are also crazy days when you just can't stick to your schedule. You can also eat meals a little later, but don't skip them completely so as not to upset your metabolism.

Indicate the portions of food you will consume at each meal.:

Stock up on the food you need

Your cupboards and refrigerator should have all the ingredients
you need for your meal plans. It is a good idea to buy all the
food you need weekly. You can freeze some foods; Save the
rest and the vegetables won't have time to spoil. A later chapter
will provide you with some sample meal plans to guide you.
Remember, you should follow your chosen plan for at least
four weeks before alternating high and low carb days.

Stock up on healthy, long-lasting carbohydrates

Many healthy carbohydrates, such as potatoes, nuts and
legumes, have a long shelf life. Buy them in bulk so you never
run out of carbs.

Recommended food portions

In addition to calorie intake and grams, the recommended
amounts of carbohydrates, some meal plans also include
half-cup or cup servings (if you use meal plans you found
online, for example). This is completely correct. No
complicated conversions required.

Keep in mind that on low carb days, your fat and protein intake will be higher. Make sure you eat healthy fats and proteins. Invest in a small food scale that allows you to easily measure grams and ounces. portions.

The recommended daily intake of carbohydrates, proteins and fats applies.

HIGH CARBOHYDRATE DAYS

TYPE OF FOOD

GRAM

BY

pound

OF

BODY WEIGHT

carbohydrates

2 – 2.5g.

Proteins

1g.

Fats

0 -0.15 g.-

LOW CARBOHYDRATE DAYS

TYPE OF FOOD

GRAM

BY

BODY

WEIGHT

carbohydrates

0.5g.

Proteins

1.5g

Fats

0.35

Once you have these basics in place, you'll be ready for the

next step.

Chapter 6: Meal Planning and Recipes

introduction

Carb cycling is a nutritional approach in which you alternate your carbohydrate intake on a daily, weekly, or monthly basis. It is often used to lose fat, maintain physical performance during a diet, or overcome a weight loss plateau.

Understand the carbohydrate cycle

When carb cycling, there are high carb days, moderate carb days, and low carb days. The idea is to reap the benefits of a high- and low-carb diet while minimizing the downsides.

High Carb Days: These days are typically scheduled around your most intense training days and allow for muscle growth and performance.

Moderate Carb Days: These generally occur on typical training days and give you enough carbs to complete your workout.

Low Carb Days: These days are typically rest days or low intensity days and help with fat loss and insulin sensitivity.

Meal planning

When planning meals for carb cycling, a balance of macronutrients is necessary. Here is a general guideline:

High carb days: 60% carbs, 25% protein, 15% fat

Moderate carb days: 40% carbs, 30% protein, 30% fat

Low carb days: 25% carbs, 40% protein, 35% fat

Please note that these percentages are only a starting point and can be adjusted based on individual needs and goals.

Recipes

Here are some recipe ideas for each type of day:

High carb day

Breakfast: Oatmeal with fruits and honey. Lunch: Quinoa salad with lots of vegetables and roast chicken. Dinner: Brown rice with roasted salmon and a side of sweet potatoes.

Moderate carb day

Breakfast: Greek yogurt with a handful of granola and red berries. Lunch: Turkey wrap with whole wheat tortilla and salad. Dinner: Grilled chicken with a side of roasted vegetables and a small portion of pasta.

Low carb day

Breakfast: Scrambled eggs with spinach and cheese. Lunch: Grilled chicken salad with lots of vegetables. Dinner: Steak with a side of asparagus and half an avocado.

Diploma

When used correctly, carb cycling can be a powerful tool. It allows for a more flexible diet and can help overcome weight loss plateaus. Remember that the most important part of any diet is its compliance. Find a routine that works for you and maintain it.Have fun on your bike!

Remember that it is always important to consult a doctor or registered dietitian before starting any new diet plan. This information is intended as general advice and may not suit everyone's nutritional needs or goals.

- Sample recipes for carb cycling days.

Example Recipes for Carb Cycling

Here are some examples of recipes for high and low carb days:

Recipes for a day rich in carbohydrates

Quinoa salad: Cooked quinoa tossed with diced vegetables, chickpeas, and a light vinaigrette dressing. This meal is rich in carbohydrates and full of protein.

Whole wheat pasta with tomato sauce: Whole wheat pasta is a good source of complex carbohydrates. Add a tomato-based sauce to lean meats or legumes for protein.

Daily low carb recipes

Grilled Chicken with Steamed Vegetables – A simple grilled chicken breast served with steamed non-starchy vegetables like broccoli, spinach, or zucchini.

Egg and Avocado Salad: Hard-boiled eggs and avocado provide a meal high in protein, high in fat, and low in carbohydrates.

Remember, the key to successful carb cycling is planning. Be sure to prepare meals that fit your high and low carb days. Always consult a nutritionist or nutritionist to ensure your meal plans meet your nutritional needs.

Chapter 7: Exercise and Carb Cycling

Introduction

Carb cycling is a nutritional strategy that alternates between high and low carb days depending on your training plan and goals. This approach is increasingly popular among athletes, bodybuilders, and those looking to lose weight.

Understand the carbohydrate cycle

Carb cycling depends on a person's training plan. Days when you train more intensely consume more carbohydrates, while low-carb days occur on days when you train less intensely. The timing and amount of carbohydrates consumed in each phase vary depending on the person.

The idea behind carb cycling is that when your body consumes a limited amount of carbohydrates, it relies on fat as its main source of energy, which can be helpful for weight management, losing body fat, and increasing carbohydrate storage when carbohydrates are reintroduced. The idea is that if you think strategically about when and how you consume carbohydrates (your body's preferred energy source for training), you can make your workouts more efficient and achieve better results in both performance and body composition.

Cycling and training with carbohydrates.
Exercise plays a crucial role in your carb cycling routine. On low-carb days, exercise encourages the body to burn fat for energy. It is generally accepted that low carbohydrate intake reduces power output during high-intensity exercise. Therefore, carb cycling can be useful if you are on a low-carb diet but want to do HIIT or weightlifting training.

Carb cycling for weight loss
 Carb cycling can be a succeseful slimming when implement correctly When your body receives a limited amount of carbohydrates, it relies on fat as its main source of energy. This can be helpful for weight management and losing body fat. However, it's important to note that high-carb days can lead to weight gain if you don't exercise as much or train hard while carb cycling.

Who should try carb cycling?

Carb cycling may be helpful for endurance athletes and active people following low-carb diets. For those focusing on endurance sports such as running, cycling, and swimming, varying carbohydrate intake throughout the year (particularly reducing carbohydrate intake during high-volume preseason training) may be helpful to Maintain muscle glycogen stores and increase performance when consuming carbohydrates. again.

Diploma

Carb cycling is a powerful tool that can help you optimize your exercise performance and help you lose weight. However, it requires careful planning and consideration of your individual training plan and nutritional needs. Always consult a doctor or registered dietitian before starting a new diet or exercise program.

Remember that the key to successful weight loss is not just cutting down on carbs or calories; It's about creating a healthy, sustainable lifestyle that includes a balanced diet and regular physical activity.

- The importance of exercise.

Introduction

Exercise plays a crucial role in any diet plan and carb cycling is no exception. Not only does it help burn calories, but it also affects how your body uses the nutrients you consume. As part of carbohydrate cycling, physical exercise can help optimize the body's utilization of carbohydrates.

The role of exercise in carbohydrate cycling.

The idea is to adapt your carbohydrate intake to your level of physical activity. On days when you exercise more (high-intensity training), you consume more carbohydrates (high-carb days). On rest days or low training intensity days, you consume fewer carbohydrates (low-carb days).

High carb days

On high-carb days, increasing your carb intake provides the fuel you need for your training. Carbohydrates are broken down into glucose, which is used to produce energy in the form of ATP (adenosine triphosphate). This energy fuels your muscles during exercise and allows you to perform at your best.

Low carb days

On low carb days, your body is forced to use fat as its main source of energy because the supply of carbohydrates is low. This can promote fat loss, which is often the goal of carb cycling. Exercise these days is usually less intense, but it is still important because it helps maintain muscle mass and metabolic health.

Exercise and metabolic flexibility.

One of the main benefits of combining exercise and carb cycling is increased metabolic flexibility. This is the body's ability to efficiently switch between burning carbohydrates and fat for energy. Regular exercise increases this flexibility and makes carb cycling more effective.

Exercise and insulin sensitivity.

Exercise also improves insulin sensitivity, which is beneficial for carbohydrate cycling. Improving insulin sensitivity allows the body to process carbohydrates better, meaning less insulin is needed to transport glucose to cells. This can result in less fat storage and more energy for your workouts.

Diploma

In short, exercise is an essential part of carbohydrate cycling. Not only does it help burn calories, but it also improves metabolic flexibility and insulin sensitivity, making the diet more effective. Whether it's a high-intensity workout on a high-carb day or a light workout on a low-carb day, staying active is key to reaping the benefits of carb cycling. Remember that a balanced approach to diet and exercise is always the best strategy to achieve your health and fitness goals.

Carb cycling for Sustainable Weight Loss
flexibility

Carb cycling is more flexible than many other diet plans. You can tailor your carbohydrate intake to your daily activity level and won't feel deprived on days when you need more energy.

Overcome stagnations

Carb cycling can help overcome weight loss plateaus. By varying your carbohydrate intake, you keep your metabolism in check, which can cause it to speed up and burn fat.

Muscle preservation

By combining high-carb days with intense workouts, you provide your body with the energy it needs to build and maintain muscle mass. This is important for long-term weight loss because muscle burns more calories than fat.

Improved hormonal balance

Carb cycling can help balance hormones associated with hunger, weight loss, and energy levels. Carb-rich days help increase levels of leptin (the "satiety hormone"), which can keep hunger at bay and improve mood. Low-carb days can lower insulin levels, which can promote fat burning.

In short, carb cycling can be a sustainable and effective way to lose weight. It provides flexibility, helps overcome weight loss plateaus, maintains muscle mass and improves hormonal balance. However, it is important to note that carb cycling should be tailored to individual needs and lifestyle. Always consult a doctor or registered dietitian before starting a new diet plan. Remember that the key to sustainable weight loss is a balanced diet combined with regular exercise.

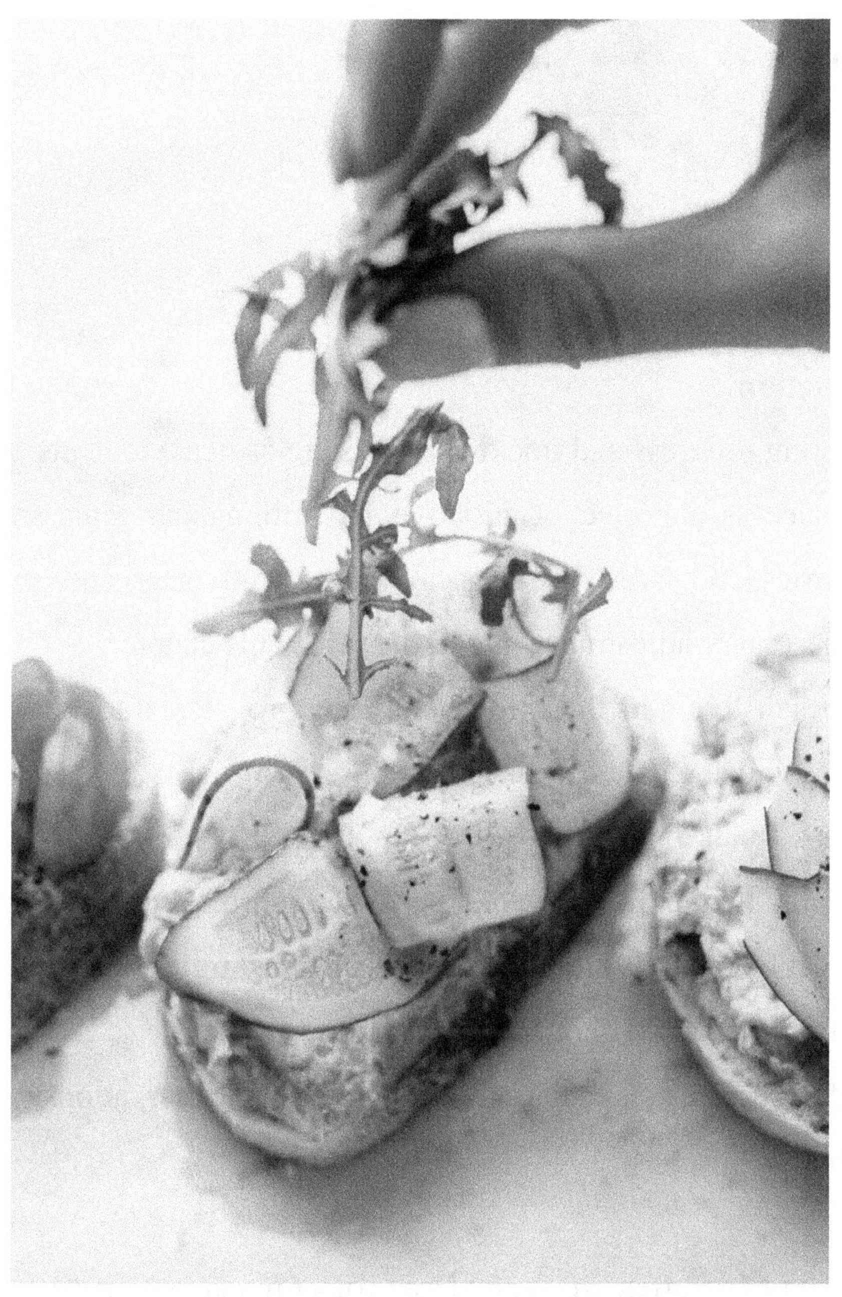

Chapter 8: Monitoring Progress and Tracking Results

introduction

Monitoring progress and tracking results are critical elements of any successful project or initiative. By setting clear goals and metrics, companies can measure their effectiveness and make necessary adjustments along the way. This chapter examines different methods for monitoring progress, tracking results, and using data to make decisions.

Progress Tracking Methods

1. **Periodic Reporting**: Creating periodic reporting schedules (e.g. weekly, monthly) to track progress against milestones and deliverables. Reports should contain both quantitative (e.g. numbers, percentages) and qualitative data (e.g. observations, comments).

2. **Project Management Tools**: Use project management software or apps (e.g. Jira, Asana) to track progress, assign tasks, and collaborate with team members. These tools

typically offer features like Gantt charts, progress timelines, and real-time updates.

3. **Key Performance Indicators (KPIs):** Define specific KPIs that measure critical aspects of the project or initiative. KPIs must be quantifiable, relevant, executable and allow for easy monitoring and evaluation. Examples of this include customer satisfaction scores, sales achieved, or employee engagement.

4. **Regular Meetings**: Hold regular team meetings to review progress, discuss challenges, and make decisions. These meetings provide an opportunity for open communication and ensure that everyone involved is on the same page.

5. **Performance Reviews**: Conduct performance reviews with team members to evaluate progress, provide feedback, and identify opportunities for improvement. This helps maintain accountability and promotes continuous learning within the team.

Tracking results

1. **Data Collection**: Collect relevant data from multiple sources (e.g. surveys, analytics, customer feedback) to measure results and evaluate impact. Data must be accurate, reliable and aligned with defined KPIs.

2. **Data Analysis**: Use statistical tools and techniques to analyze data, identify trends, and draw meaningful conclusions. This may include using dashboards, spreadsheets, or specialized software to process and interpret data.

3. **Reports and visualization**: Present results in clear and concise reports and visualizations (e.g., charts, graphs, infographics). This makes it easier to understand the results and allows decision makers to take informed action.

Use data to make decisions

1. **Evidence-based decisions**:   Use data to support decision-making processes to ensure that decisions are based on objective information rather than assumptions or biases.

2. **Continuous improvement**: Analyze data to identify
areas for improvement, develop strategies, and make necessary
adjustments to increase effectiveness.

3. **Performance Optimization**: Using data to optimize
performance, identify bottlenecks and implement solutions to
maximize production and achieve better results.

4. **Early warning system**: Monitoring data can act as an
early warning system, allowing companies to identify potential
problems or risks early and take preventative measures.

5. **Resource Allocation**: Use data to justify resource
allocation decisions to ensure resources are directed to areas
with the greatest potential for impact.

Challenges and Considerations

1. **Data integrity**: Ensure the accuracy and reliability of
data used for monitoring and tracking. This requires rigorous
data collection and validation processes.

2. **Data Interpretation**:   Interpret data correctly and avoid misinterpretation or bias. Involving experts or consulting with statisticians can help conduct a proper analysis.

3. **Timeliness**:   Ensure data is collected and analyzed in a timely manner to support decision making and avoid delays.

4. **Communication**:   Communicate results effectively, clearly and practically to interested parties to facilitate understanding and drive appropriate action.

Chapter 9: Common Questions and Concerns

1. **Is carb cycling effective for weight loss**?

Yes, carb cycling can be an effective way to lose weight, but it's not a miracle cure. It's important to combine carb cycling with a healthy diet and regular exercise for optimal results.

2. **Is carb cycling safe**?

Carb cycling is generally safe for healthy adults. However, it's not recommended for people with certain medical conditions, such as diabetes or kidney disease. It's always a good idea to talk to your doctor before starting any new diet.

3. **Will carb cycling make me lose muscle**?

Carb cycling can help you preserve muscle mass, especially when combined with resistance training. However, it's important to make sure you're getting enough protein and calories overall.

4. **How often should I cycle carbs?**

The frequency of carb cycling depends on your individual needs and goals. Some people cycle carbs every day, while others cycle them every 2-3 days or even weekly.

5. **What types of foods should I eat on high-carb days?**

On high-carb days, focus on eating nutrient-rich foods such as whole grains, fruits, vegetables, and lean protein.

6. **What types of foods should I eat on low-carb days?**

On low-carb days, limit your intake of carbohydrates and focus on eating healthy fats and protein. Good choices include lean meats, fish, eggs, nuts, seeds, and non-starchy vegetables.

7. **How long can I stay on a carb cycling diet?**

Carb cycling can be a long-term lifestyle approach to weight loss and maintenance. However, it's important to listen to your body and make adjustments as needed.

8. **Are there any side effects of carb cycling?**

Some people may experience side effects such as fatigue, headaches, and muscle cramps when first starting carb cycling. These side effects typically subside within a few days or weeks.

9. **Is carb cycling a good option for everyone**?

Carb cycling may not be suitable for everyone. This offering is not deemed suitable for individuals grappling with specific health concerns. Additionally, those with a history of disruptive eating patterns may find alternative approaches more appropriate.

*10. **How do I know if carb cycling is working for me?**

You should start to see results within a few weeks of starting carb cycling.

- Addressing FAQs about Carb Cycling

Q: What is carb cycling?

A: Carb cycling is a diet approach where carbohydrate intake is varied throughout the week. High-carb days are typically followed by low-carb days or no-carb days.

Q: What are the benefits of carb cycling?

A: **Carb cycling may help**:

* Improve body composition by reducing body fat and preserving muscle
* Enhance athletic performance by providing energy for glycogen stores
* Boost metabolism by increasing thermogenesis
* Reduce insulin resistance

Q: What are the potential risks of carb cycling?

A: **Potential risks include**:

* Electrolyte imbalances, especially during low-carb periods
* Dehydration
* Macronutrient deficiencies if the diet is not well-balanced
* Fatigue and irritability on low-carb days

Q: **Who is carb cycling suitable for?**

A: **Carb cycling may be appropriate for:**

* Advanced athletes who need to manipulate glycogen stores for optimal performance

* Individuals with insulin resistance or type 2 diabetes who want to improve blood sugar control

* Those looking to improve body composition

Q: How to implement carb cycling?

A: Carb cycling protocols vary, but a common approach is:

*   **High-carb day**:   4-6 grams of carbs per kilogram of body weight

*   **Medium-carb day**:   2-3 grams of carbs per kilogram of body weight

*   **Low-carb day**:   0-1 gram of carbs per kilogram of body weight

Q: Is carb cycling sustainable?

A: Carb cycling can be sustainable if it is tailored to individual needs and goals. It is important to periodize the diet and gradually transition from one phase to another.

Q: How long should I carb cycle for?

A: The duration of a carb cycling cycle can vary from a few weeks to several months.

Seek the expertise of a qualified registered dietitian or healthcare provider to ensure tailored guidance and avoid potential risks.

Q: Should I consult a healthcare professional before starting carb cycling?

A: Yes, it is highly recommended to consult with a healthcare professional, especially if you have any underlying health conditions or if you are new to carb cycling.

– Dealing with Challenges and Misconceptions

Dealing with Challenges and Misconceptions about Carb Cycling

Challenges:

* **Difficulty in calculating macronutrient ratios**: Determining the optimal ratios for individual needs can be complex and requires precise tracking.
* **Hunger and cravings**: Reducing carbohydrates can initially lead to hunger and cravings, especially on high-carb days.
* **Electrolyte imbalances**: Carb cycling can alter electrolyte levels, requiring supplementation or careful dietary adjustments.
* **Consistency**: Maintaining a consistent cycle over time can be challenging due to social events, travel, or other factors.

Misconceptions:

* **Carb cycling is just a fad**: Carb cycling has been used by athletes and bodybuilders for decades and is supported by scientific evidence.
* **Carb cycling will lead to muscle loss:** When done correctly, carb cycling can actually promote muscle growth.

* **High-carb days will make you gain fat**: While excess calories can lead to weight gain, high-carb days are necessary to replenish muscle glycogen stores and support recovery.

* **Low-carb days will put you into ketosis:** Short-term low-carb phases do not typically lead to ketosis unless carbohydrate intake is extremely low.

Overcoming Challenges:

* **Seek professional guidance**: Consult a registered dietitian or certified personal trainer for personalized advice on macronutrient ratios and meal plans.

* **Listen to your body:** Pay attention to hunger cues and adjust calorie intake or macronutrient ratios accordingly.

* **Hydrate well**: Drink plenty of fluids, especially on high-carb days, to prevent electrolyte imbalances.

* **Be patient and consistent**: Carb cycling takes time to adjust to and results may not be immediate.

Addressing Misconceptions:

* **Provide scientific evidence**: Cite studies and research that support the benefits of carb cycling.

*   **Explain the mechanisms**:   Describe how carb cycling manipulates insulin levels and promotes muscle growth.

*   **Highlight the importance of portion control**:   Emphasize that even on high-carb days, it's crucial to eat in moderation to avoid weight gain.

*   **Clarify the definition of ketosis**:   Explain that ketosis requires very low carbohydrate intake for an extended period, which is not typically achieved through carb cycling.

Chapter 10: Conclusion and Next Steps

Carb cycling involves alternating periods of high-carb and low-carb intake to manipulate hormonal responses and energy availability. While effective for certain goals and individuals, it requires careful planning and adherence.

Key Considerations for Continuing Carb Cycling:

* **Monitor progress:** Track body composition, performance, and energy levels to assess the effectiveness of the diet.

* **Adjust macros**: Fine-tune carbohydrate intake based on individual needs and goals.

* **Hydrate adequately**: Carb cycling can lead to dehydration, so ensure adequate fluid intake.

* **Listen to the body**: Pay attention to hunger cues and adjust carb intake accordingly.

* **Maintain consistency**: Follow the prescribed cycling schedule consistently for optimal results.

* **Consider nutrient timing**: Optimize carbohydrate intake around workouts and recovery periods.

Potential Next Steps:

* **Maintain carb cycling**: Continue with the current regimen if it aligns with goals and yields desired results.

* **Transition to a different diet**: Explore alternative dietary approaches that may be more sustainable or beneficial.

* **Seek professional guidance**: Consult with a registered dietitian or healthcare professional for personalized advice and support.

Important Note: Carb cycling is not a quick fix or a cure-all. It requires a disciplined approach and long-term commitment. Individuals with underlying health conditions or dietary restrictions should consult with a healthcare professional before embarking on such a diet.

- Moving Forward with Carb Cycling for Continued Success

To continue experiencing success with carb cycling, consider the following tips:

1. **Monitor Progress and Adjust**:

* Track your progress by regularly monitoring your weight, body measurements, and energy levels.
* If you reach a plateau or experience setbacks, adjust your carb intake or cycling schedule accordingly.

2. **Experiment with Different Carb Load Amounts**:

* Determine the optimal carb load amounts for your body and goals. Experiment with varying high-carb and low-carb days.
* Pay attention to how different carb loads affect your performance, recovery, and overall well-being.

3. **Prioritize Nutrient-Rich Foods**:

* Focus on consuming nutrient-rich, whole foods during all phases of the cycle.
* Choose high-fiber vegetables, lean protein, and healthy fats to support overall health and performance.

4. **Stay Hydrated**:

* Drink plenty of water throughout the day, especially on high-carb days.
* Adequate hydration helps enhance performance, reduce fatigue, and support recovery.

5. **Listen to Your Body**:

* Listen to your body's response to Carb Cycling Adjust the frequency or duration of cycles based on your individual needs and preferences.
* If you experience extreme fatigue, headaches, or digestive issues, consider modifying your approach.

6. **Combine with Exercise**:

* Engage in regular exercise during carb cycling to maximize calorie expenditure and performance.
* Choose activities that align with your fitness goals and complement the carb cycle schedule.

7. **Consider a Nutritionist or Coach**:

* If you need personalized guidance or support, consider seeking advice from a registered dietitian or certified fitness coach.
* They can provide tailored plans and ongoing support to help you achieve your goals effectively and safely.

8. **Be Patient and Consistent**:

* Carb cycling requires patience and consistency to see optimal results.
* Stay dedicated to the plan and make gradual adjustments as needed to maintain long-term success.

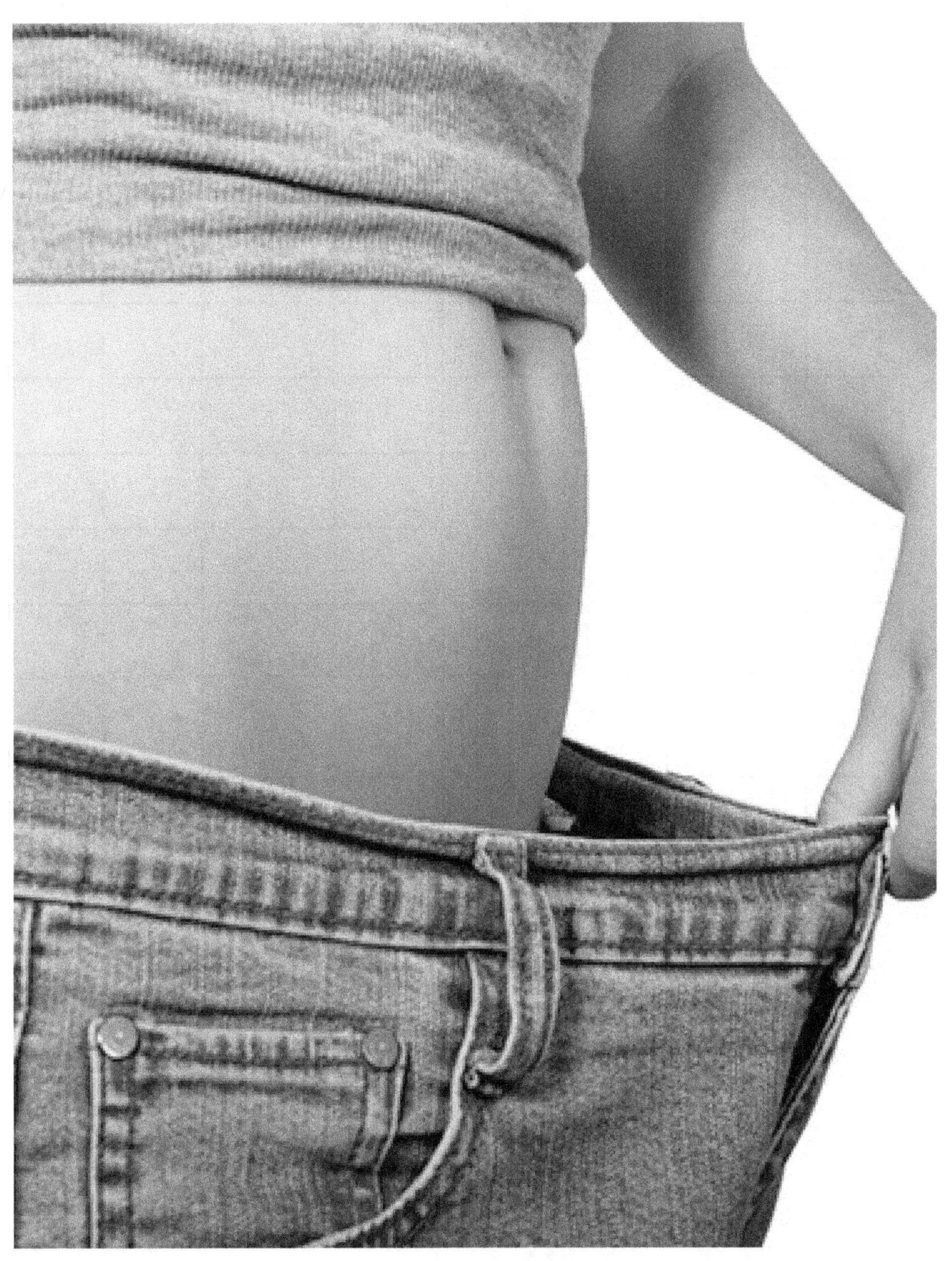

Happy Ending

Days	Low Carb Days	Low Carb Day.	High Carb Day	Low Carb Day	Low Carb Day	High Carb Day	Low Carb Day
1							
2							
.3							
4							
5							
6							
7							

www.ingramcontent.com/pod-product-compliance
Lightning Source LLC
Chambersburg PA
CBHW081600250726
48653CB00009B/3517